Why is My Child a Slow Reader and Struggling in School?

Why is My Child a Slow Reader and Struggling in School?

WHAT EVERY PARENT NEEDS TO KNOW

Michael Conte, O.D.
& Barry Fretwell, O.D.

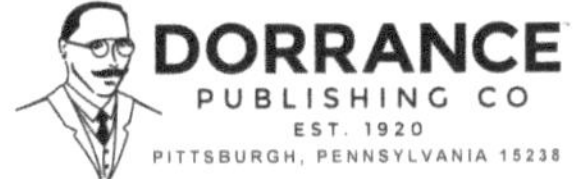

CONTENTS

Why is My Child a Slow Reader and Struggling in School?

Understanding How Vision and Vertical Phorias Impact a Child's Learning

"This homework is stupid!" Sam exclaimed, shoving the book across the table and flinging himself back in his chair.

"Well, you're not leaving that chair until it's finished," his mother replied firmly. "Your teacher says that you still haven't handed in four separate assignments. That's four zeroes, Sam."

"I don't care. I hate school," the ten-year-old responded sullenly.

"You still have to do your homework." She sighed then drew a deep breath, steeling herself for the battle to come.

Is this a familiar scene at your house? Want to change it?

Unfortunately, this scenario is all too familiar for many parents. They watch in frustration as their child falls further and further behind in school, while his self-esteem is stripped away layer by layer with every failure. Their home becomes a battleground rather than a sanctuary.

Even when parents suspect the issue may be due to a vision problem and take their child to an optometrist, often the underlying cause is misdiagnosed.

During the second half of the school year a father and son came to visit me (Michael D. Conte O.D.) for an eye exam. While the boy was already wearing glasses to help him see the blackboard better, he was still having unexplained difficulty with reading fluency and comprehension. The parents, both medical doctors, had taken their son to several professionals, including a leading pediatric ophthalmologist. It greatly relieved the parents to learn that he did not have ADD (Attention Deficit Disorder), nor was he dyslexic. Beyond that they found no answers.

Their ten-year-old complained that when he read it made him tired and that he constantly lost his place and was unable to focus on the reading material. His father wanted a second opinion as to why he was frustrated by his poor reading comprehension and his glasses didn't help.

During my examination I took particular care with the binocular evaluation, especially at the near reading position. The result showed their son had a vertical phoria and accommodation problem. Now that we had an accurate diagnosis of the child's problem, it was relatively easy to treat. The treatment consisted of new bifocal glasses with prism and a referral for vision therapy.

The results were amazing. All the initial complaints were resolved within two weeks, and the father called after four weeks to remark that for the first time his son could sit still and read for several hours; he now even enjoyed reading. He wanted to know how and why the treatment plan worked, especially since he was a pediatric doctor. I now want to answer his questions, in the hope that it will help other parents with children who suffer from the same disability.

CHAPTER 1

What Is the Relationship Between Vision, Reading, and Learning?

Just how important are proper vision and vision skills in a child's ability to learn to read and do well in school? What are the individual and socio-economic consequences of not ensuring that your child has proper vision skills early in school and throughout their development? We will look at some data in this chapter that may surprise you.

Allan Cott, MD, a psychiatrist in New York City, writes in his book, *Help for Your Learning-Disabled Child*, that he ordinarily includes an evaluation of his patients by a developmental/behavioral optometrist as part of their initial evaluation. He states:

> "An examination of a learning-disabled child without a
> consultation and treatment by a developmental optometrist
> is an incomplete examination and treatment."

As concerned parents, we all want our children to perform well in school, and having clear vision in combination with excellent vision skills are more important for a child's learning and social development than the majority of parents, teachers, and doctors realize, as you will learn in this book. We buy them new clothes, school supplies, and make sure they have a medical check-up for a new school year, but how many parents take their child to the eye doctor at the beginning of each school year for a vision exam?

Unfortunately many parents, if not most, rely on the vision screenings at school or the pediatrician's office to detect vision problems. But they are unaware that these types of vision screenings are not designed to detect vision-related problems, except for the most apparent cases such as severe nearsightedness or lazy eye. The school vision screening and the pediatrician's office screening only test clearness of sight usually at ten or twenty feet, and are not intended to replace a through, professional eye exam by an eye doctor. The earlier a vision-related difficulty is detected and treated, the better chance a child has to respond well to treatment and proper development of other skills related to vision, such as reading and a classroom work.

From grade school through college, a student's visual system must meet high demands; both, for instance, vision and near focusing for reading. No task is more challenging in the early years than learning to read and reading to learn. Learning to read and reading to learn are truly the fundamental building blocks of doing well in school and in many other areas of life.

It is estimated that 20-25 percent of school-aged children have serious difficulty with reading, which is near epidemic levels.

Too many of these children will pass the school vision screening test, be told they have normal vision by the school nurse, and end up being diagnosed as having a learning disability, being a slow learner, having dyslexia, or having ADD because they have trouble with their near vision but not their distance vision. Sadly, it is rare that someone in the educational system will be knowledgeable enough to refer these children for a comprehensive eye exam, which includes perception skills and binocular testing, and so the child is placed in remedial learning programs.

When 35 percent of the population is affected by a treatable disability, it may be considered by some to be an epidemic. When that disability is the leading cause of emotional problems in children and adolescents in North America, we are talking about a serious public health problem. Such a large number of school-aged children having serious difficulty with reading results in not only poor performance in school but also detrimental behavioral and social and economic consequences through-out their life.

Consider that this near epidemic number of 20-25 percent is a major contributing factor in school dropouts and juvenile delinquency. Carl L. Kline, a child and adolescent psychiatrist internationally known for his expertise in children's learning disabilities states, "Although a definitive study has not yet been done, it seems likely that teenagers who can't read or spell and who consequently hate school are easy targets for drug dealers."

Reading and learning requires children to use all their language and decoding skills, and the coordination of three aspects of the visual system must be working correctly: visual acuity, visual cognitive processing and visual efficacy. Your optometrist's first area of concern is with correcting visual acuity (clearness of sight) and testing for the monocular (function of one eye) and binocular visual (both eyes working together) skills and capabilities at both distances near and far. Visual cognitive processing depends in a large part not only on the clearness of vision at distances both near and far but also on psychological and intellectual development, prior experience, visual memory, and motivation. Visual efficacy, or the ability to achieve the desired results of learning with good self-esteem, depends on combining sharp vision and proper eye motor control skills with intellectual capacity.

Research shows that children who read well in the early grades are far more successful in later years; and those who fall behind often stay behind when it comes to academic achievement.

It is estimated by most educators that approximately 80-90 percent of classroom learning is attributed to vision; it is no surprise that poor vision or poor vision skills result in poor attention and poor learning. Poor vision impacting learning development and behavior problems during early childhood may well explain the association between the lack of academic achievement, antisocial behavior, and delinquency. For example, numerous studies have shown that delinquents' verbal IQs tend to be lower than their nonverbal IQs (e.g., Moffitt, 1993). Delinquents also have lower mean global IQs and lower school achievement rates compared with non-delinquents.

A study by Dennis Hogenson, *Reading Failure and Juvenile Delinquency*, is remarkable both in what it found and what it didn't find: "...the present study was unsuccessful in attempting to correlate aggression with age, family size, or number of parents present in the home, rural versus urban environment, socio-economic status, minority group membership, religious preference, etc." The surprising outcome is that only reading failure was found to correlate with aggression in delinquent boys.

"It is possible that reading failure is the single most significant factor in those forms of delinquency which can be described as anti-socially aggressive. I am speaking of assault, arson, sadistic acts directed against peers and siblings, major vandalism, etc.," said Hogenson.

For too long being poor or coming from a poor neighborhood was reported widely to be the cause for illiteracy, juvenile delinquency, and anti-social behavior, but this is not true. A Cincinnati newspaper headline said it best: "Poor black students disproving myths." The article states, "Washburn's students scored higher than many other in the Cincinnati Public School system....They rank near the top among city schools in writing ability..." The principal noted that "[s]ome of the students come to school without breakfast, and lack adequate clothing" and that "97 percent of them receive some type of public assistance." Washburn is located in a high drug area in the "low-income West End" of Cincinnati.

These astonishing facts bring the magnitude of our country's need for more attention by educators, parents, and politicians, to encourage and/or provide proper comprehensive vision examinations by a qualified eye doctor in children's vision clearness and vision perceptual skills at the beginning of each school year. Without question, good vision and visual skills are absolutely necessary for quality learning of children in America.

Additional data presented below helps bring into focus how important proper vision skills, learning to read, and reading to learn affects our society. Although the cause of juvenile delinquency and crime are known to be multifactorial: individual, family, peer, school, and community, we think proper vision and vision skills may be much more important early in life than the attention it is currently given.

1. More than ten million children in the U.S. have vision problems that may contribute to poor academic performance, according to the National Parent Teacher Association. Up to 85 percent of both Title I students in the fifth through eighth grades and academically as well as behaviorally at-risk children between the ages of eight and eighteen have vision problems that are either undetected or untreated.

2. Teenagers who have low SAT scores and mediocre academic records have a high incidence of undetected or untreated vision problems. Such students are at risk for not completing a college education. In addition, uncorrected vision problems have been linked to high school drop-out rates.

3. A shocking 85 percent of all juveniles who interface with the juvenile court system are functionally illiterate.

4. Illiteracy and crime are closely related. The Department of Justice states, "The link between academic failure and delinquency, violence, and crime is welded to reading failure." Over 70 percent of inmates in America's prisons cannot read above a fourth grade level.

5. The health care industry estimates $73 billion per year of unnecessary health care expenses attributable to poor literacy. One in three adults cannot read this sentence.

6. Two-thirds of children in the United States do not receive any preventive vision care before entering elementary school. Once children enter school the problem only gets worse.

It's easy to understand that we have a huge problem in our nation due to poor vision, poor reading ability, and poor learning starting early in life and negatively affecting the individual's life and our entire society, both in lost personal productivity and self-esteem as well as a huge cost to our nation.

In order to reverse this disturbing trend in the U.S., we recommend that all children are not only taken to their pediatrician at an early age for their medical checkup but also to an optometrist or ophthalmologist for an eye/vision examination to determine if vision correction is needed and if a medical condition or binocular/perception error exists that would prevent a child from having the best visual capabilities possible for learning.

If, however, a child who has had the basic vision examination and is said to be normal but continues to have the same problematic symptoms with reading and comprehension in school after all other conditions such as medical, psychological, and vision clearness are corrected or ruled out, you should seek the help of a developmental or behavioral optometrist who specializes in binocular vision diagnosis and treatment, prior to having the child labeled as learning disabled, dyslexic, having ADD, and having psychoactive drugs prescribed. Don't make the mistake of assuming that just because you are told your child has 20/20 vision everything is all right. This may not be true.

There are numerous visual, psychological, and medically related conditions that can affect children's reading, learning, and comprehension skills. We are intentionally directing our primary discussion in the following chapters on one visual diagnosis that is more often than not overlooked by eye doctors when examining students with complaints of poor reading and school performance.

All optometrists and ophthalmologists are trained to examine for the common vision problems such as refractive and medical defects at all eye examinations. These include external and internal pathology, myopia, hyperopia, astigmatism, and accommodation, as well as other tests. Most optometrists and ophthalmologists agree to have a child's first eye exam not later than in the fourth year, sooner if you observe or suspect eye problems, followed by yearly visits to the eye doctor.

Again, many parents and general medical doctors are not aware that school vision screenings are not intended to substitute for the eye doctor's exams yearly, nor will school vision screenings uncover any but the most apparent vision problems. School vision screenings are set up to only test the eyes at a distance (ten feet in Texas), but do not test a child's ability to read at a near distance, his focusing ability, his eye alignment, or his eye coordination.

Parents tell us all the time that their child's last eye exam was at school, incorrectly assuming everything was tested. Therefore, school screenings actually give parents the false impression that their child has no vision problems, and their child's struggling with schoolwork is not related to vision.

This book will not attempt to cover every vision disorder that will result in poor school performance and poor learning ability; other books are already available which do an excellent job with that. This book is intended to help educate the public about one specific binocular visual condition that is most often forgotten by the vast majority of eye care specialist; this condition directly interferes with reading and learning ability if not detected and corrected. We will focus our main discussion to a binocular condition known as *vertical phoria*, which is only one condition out of many which can directly impact a child's reading and learning ability.

We hope the information presented in this book will result in parents, educators, fellow doctors and politicians being more aware of the need for early professional vision care. Eye specialists who have the knowledge of binocular problems such as vertical phoria symptoms are extremely important in the evaluation, diagnosis, and treatment of school- aged children. This information is especially important for parents who have children that are struggling with reading, math, learning, and schoolwork after being told their child's vision is 20/20. Even college students and adults with difficulty reading will benefit if this condition is found to be present and is corrected.

What is a vertical phoria? Vertical phoria is a binocular condition in which the eyes are not in perfect alignment in the vertical direction, meaning one eye is slightly higher than the other and they do not work together perfectly when reading.

This condition should be high on the suspected vision problem list in determining the cause and treatment of any person complaining of any or all of the following: headaches, tired eyes, poor concentration, and poor reading skills, as well as motion sickness. The presence of a vertical phoria directly impacts math, reading, and learning skills, especially important in school-aged children and can cause motion sickness.

Current literature suggest that 9-15 percent of the population in the U.S. is estimated to have a vertical phoria; that's as high as seventy-five in a group of five hundred students, or as many as over forty million people in the United States. Since approximately 80-90 percent or of all academic learning in school is related to vision, it's easy to understand that if a child's visual system is not functioning properly they will be at a huge disadvantage academically. With this book we hope to get the word out that there is help for many of these children and that you can avoid any unnecessary labeling or stigma being placed on any child that has normal intelligence and abilities but has trouble in school due to undiagnosed vision difficulties.

Educators, school nurses, fellow doctors, and parents who see students who are having difficulty reading and keeping up in school should make an appointment with a developmental or behavioral optometrist prior to treatment with the Irene Color Overlay Program, Bridges Learning Program, labeling the child with dyslexia, learning disability, Attention Deficit Hyperactive Disorder (ADHD), or prescribing behavior modification drugs. Children may still need and benefit from these therapies and/or medication, but the clearness of vision at distance as well as near, oculomotor and visual skills should be examined first by an optometrist who is knowledgeable about binocular, accommodative, and vertical phoria testing and correction.

You may find a local developmental or behavioral optometrist at *http://www.covd.org*. If you do not have a College of Optometrists in Visual Developmental (COVD) optometrist nearby, we recommend that you phone your local optometrist and ask if they test for binocular function during an eye exam and if they can provide vision therapy if needed. Ask specifically if they test for the presence of a vertical phoria. Should they not be familiar with vertical phoria, call another optometrist. COVD certification is not required for an optometrist to be alert and competent to diagnose and treat vertical phoria, as well as all other vision-related issues.

All optometrists and ophthalmologists have exposure to this visual anomaly in their professional training, but it seems it is too often forgotten in practice. As a matter of fact, you should understand that not all optometrists and ophthalmologists think it is important to test a child for vertical phoria, other eye alignment issues, or eye co-ordination function. They are under the false impression that these issues have no impact on learning abilities of a child in the classroom. The lack of attention to correcting this condition is due in large part to lack of awareness by the general public and school teachers, and in other cases where individual doctors have a personal preconception that there is no need to test for or correct what they consider small amounts of vertical phoria. Instead they stop the eye exam once clearness of vision is present either with or without corrective eyewear. Unfortunately, this results in leaving too many parents and children with an incorrect diagnosis of being a slow reader, learning disabled, or having ADHD because they are frustrated while trying to read after they are told nothing is wrong with their vision.

CHAPTER 2

What is the Association Between Developmental Vision and Learning?

It may surprise many parents, teachers, and educators to find out that many of these children having trouble in school actually have vision problems as the root of their difficulties. According to the National PTA, "It is estimated that more than ten million children (ages 0-10) suffer from vision problems that may cause them to fail in school."

Don't be lulled into thinking that because a child sees an eye chart across the room clearly that he or she has perfect vision. "Twenty/twenty" is simply the ability to see at twenty feet what a person with normal vision should be able to see on an eye chart at twenty feet.

First, to understand why the child in our opening example is having so much trouble and dislikes reading, we need to review the fundamentals involved in vision and learning. Vision is learned. From our earliest moments in life, we develop our ability to use sight to match up information with our mobility and other senses to integrate, organize, confirm, and develop experience to relate to our environment. This is vision.

The experience of vision is considered the primary means by which the child or adult explores and understands their environment. Vision also becomes a primary influence in higher functions such as attention, concentration, comprehension, and especially learning.

To help in understanding some of the visual skills required for school-work, think about the classroom environment. A child sits at a desk, writes, alternately reads from a textbook and from the chalkboard, and usually follows the teacher's movements around the room while listening to the lesson. Some of the visual skills required in the classroom are:

1. *Distance vision:* being able to see the board clearly.

2. *Near vision:* being able to see the word in a book clearly.

3. *Focusing flexibility:* being able to maintain clear vision while changing focus from a distant object to a near object.

4. *Tracking/eye movement skills:* being able to align both eyes accurately and move smoothly together across a line of print or from object to object with ease.

5. *Eye-hand coordination:* being able to use the eyes to guide the hands.

6. *Eye teaming:* being able to coordinate the two eyes together so that they are precisely directed at the same object at the same time.

7. *Eye focusing:* maintaining, for long periods of time, completely clear vision while looking at near or distant objects.

Students who have eye teaming, tracking, and focusing deficiencies often have complaints of losing their place while reading, tired eyes, trouble focusing, dizziness, nausea, headaches, and/or red, burning, and itchy eyes. They usually occur after the student is required to maintain visual concentration; for example, doing a reading lesson is enough to stress a student's visual system when it is deficient in any of the above skills and may cause fatigue, restlessness, and difficulty paying attention.

A study at the University of California in San Diego has recently pointed toward a link between ADHD and vision disorders. One of the concerns raised by this study is that untreated vision trouble causes symptoms that may easily be mistaken for ADHD.

Children lacking these visual skills may not report symptoms even though they may tire easily, see double, or have "ghost images" at times while reading for long periods. Their schoolwork may be poor, or they may not be reaching their full potential. It is not uncommon for these children to have difficulty with reading, math, paying attention, or even to exhibit behavioral problems in the classroom. Since these are also symptoms of ADHD, it is easy to understand how easily one could be mistaken for the other.

"We have shown that children with convergence insufficiency (difficulty focusing both eyes at a target and getting a clear single image) are three times as likely to be diagnosed as having ADHD as children without this visual disorder", says David B. Granet, MD, a UCSD School of Medicine professor of Ophthalmology and Pediatrics and also Director of the UCSD Ratner Children's Eye Center. One of the possible reasons for this connection given by Dr. Granet is that sometimes these vision problems are being misdiagnosed as ADHD. Convergence insufficiency "makes it more difficult to concentrate on reading, which is also one of the ways doctors diagnosed ADHD," Dr. Granet commented.

This new research appears to support what developmental optometrists have been saying for many years. There are numerous optometric studies showing a close connection between vision and learning. In fact, some studies have shown that a significant percentage of children with learning disabilities have some type of learning-related vision difficulty.

Children such as the one discussed in the introduction often have undiagnosed vision and visual skills issues that directly interfere with learning abilities in the classroom, even though they have been told they can see 20/20 on a vision screening test. You now know that frequently these vision problems are not detected during a routine doctor's office eye screening or school vision screening by a nurse. The ability of a child to read the 20/20 letters on a wall chart in no way ensures they have the proper vision or visual skills for their success in school which involves distance and near vision skills needed in the classroom.

These well-known facts concerning the link between the quality of vision and vision skills directly impacting the ability of a child to be successful in school is knowledge that has been understood for over forty years by vision care specialists. Regrettably, this information continues to be poorly received by most medical eye practitioners, many optometric practitioners, and academic professionals, resulting in no largely organized national effort to eliminate failures and dropouts in our schools due to vision-related learning issues.

We have learned that an estimated 80-90 percent of classroom learning comes by way of vision. So it's easy to understand that any child with an undiagnosed vision problem will not do well in school, seem to have a short attention span, become disruptive, and could possibly be incorrectly labeled as a slow learner, dyslexic, having ADHD, or being learning disabled.

Although it makes little sense to only screen visual clearness at distance and then to send the child back to the classroom to work for the next several hours performing reading and writing tasks at near, this is presently the standard that is being used in schools across the United States. Elementary school nurses are known to pass a child on the eye chart screening test if they can read no better than the 20/40 line of letters at a distance, while never testing near vision. This practice does not serve our children, parents, or the futures of our children well.

Keep in mind that there are numerous subtle vision errors that may exist and are unrelated to the ability to read 20/20 letters on an eye chart, which are important to identify during a vision screening or yearly eye exam by an eye specialist. Functional, medical, behavioral, emotional, and/or developmental vision problems can also cause interference with the ability to do well with reading and learning in school, even when the child can read the 20/20 letters at distance and near.

If eyes are not working together properly, children will have difficulty maintaining their eyes in alignment, particularly when reading and writing. Vision problems with near focusing can also interfere with a child's ability to maintain visual attention during reading and writing activities, as well as when focusing from the board back to their desk work.

Uncorrected visual skills, that a behavioral/developmental optometrist specializes in detecting and treating will interfere with the ability of a child to concentrate in school and result in frustration both for the child, teacher, and parent. Poor vision and vision skills many times lead to impaired perceptual abilities and may even cause failure in academic grades, social development, and developmental delays.

To have your child examined for visual skills beyond a routine eye exam, you should seek a behavioral/developmental vision specialist, which refers to an eye doctor who has the practice emphasis and educational background to understand, diagnose, and treat vision problems that are not only functional (ability to see an eye chart clearly, normal eye muscle coordination, etc.), but also problems of visual processing and integration of visual skills. Any deficiencies in these areas directly affect the ability to attend, concentrate, and orient ourselves in our spatial world and especially with regarding and learning. A behavioral vision eye exam differs from a routine eye examination since the doctor will do additional testing and spend time analyzing eye coordination, perception, and vision behavior to gain more information about any visual inequities.

Eye doctors performing standard eye examinations often miss the functional and perceptual vision problems that are essential in near vision activities. It is not uncommon that after a standard eye examination is performed, the eye doctor will inform the parents that the child has healthy eyes and that the vision is normal, or 20/20, which leaves parents incorrectly thinking poor performance in school is not related to the vision.

Unfortunately, some eye doctors will frequently not test for convergence, vertical phoria, horizontal phoria, or near focusing ability. The lack of these vision skills generally relate to symptoms of eye strain, headaches, reading problems, reduced comprehension, poor attention span, disruptive behavior, and learning difficulties.

A vision examination should include a careful functional analysis of not only perceptual vision complaints, but also near vision skills such as the ability to develop pursuit tracking saccades (quick eye movements), to change focus quickly, and to sustain focusing ability. To give children the highest potential for achievement and academic advancement, parents should seek 20/20 vision plus these other vision skills to rule out any functional or perceptual vision issues. Next we will explain in more detail what a vertical phoria is.

A study at the University of California in San Diego has recently pointed toward a link between ADHD and vision problems. One of the concerns raised by this study is that the vision problem causes symptom that could easily be mistaken for ADHD. This new research appears to support what developmental optometrists have been saying for many years.

The idea of vision problems interfering with school performance is gaining momentum with national organizations. The National PTA voiced concern that "the relationship between poorly developed visual skills and poor academic performance is not widely held among students, parents, teachers, school administrators, and public health officials" and actually passed a resolution stating that the "National PTA, through its constituent organizations, provides information to educate members, educators, administrators, public health officials, and the public at large about learning related visual problems." Consequently, we know there is a very important link between a child's proper vision and vision skills associated with classroom learning, behavior, and even long-term life achievement.

CHAPTER 3

Vertical Phoria:
The Forgotten Diagnosis

Now let's concentrate our attention on the more specific visual disorder of vertical phoria, which, you are now aware, directly impacts reading and learning ability but is by and large never tested for in children by the majority of eye care providers. We routinely examine children in our office, who are doing poorly in school, are wearing glasses that have been recently prescribed elsewhere, and do correct the child to 20/20 vision, but the child is one or more grade levels behind in reading and struggling in school.

So, what is a vertical phoria?

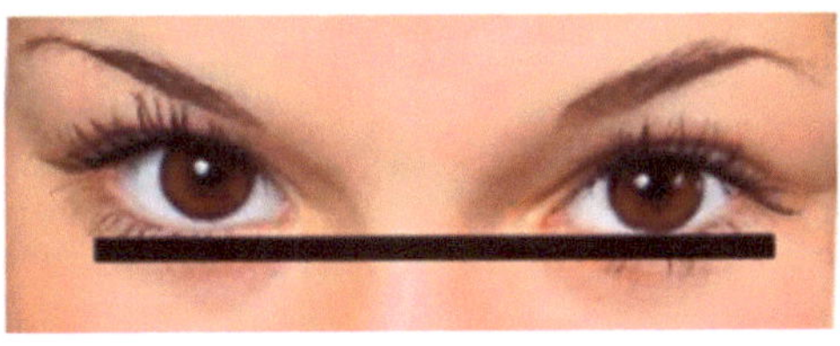

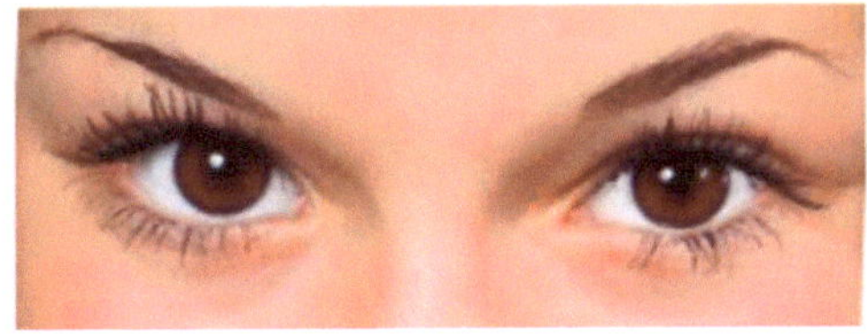

It has been said that a picture is worth a thousand words. The first picture above shows how the eyes are not vertically aligned. The picture shows the right eye hyper (higher) in relation to the left eye. This image illustrates a vertical phoria that is easy to see. Keep this picture in mind as we go along. This person will have to tilt their head to the right side in order for the eyes to be on the same plain. Generally patients have such a small deviation in alignment of the visual axis that it is undetectable by simple observation by the patient or other individuals This is illustrated by the second picture and is not as easy to see the right hyper, yet both individuals will have symptoms directly associated with vertical phoria, which we will describe later.

Vertical phoria is a condition involving an ocular neuromuscular imbalance between the two eyes which affects the ability to maintain fixation in the vertical plane when re-fixating on different points or objects during any activity involving the eyes while in dynamic use such as reading.

That is to say, it is when the visual axis or fixation of the two eyes does not align in the vertical perfectly without some adjustment such as a head tilt. This failure to re-fixate when reading from the end of one line to the next is the very reason children have to use their finger or some kind of visual aid that helps them stay on the correct line. These children are slow readers with reduced comprehension. A vertical phoria may be present in children, as well as adults. Individuals may suffer symptoms from a vertical phoria at distance viewing only, near viewing only, or both distance and near viewing. Commonly, it is genetically transmitted to children by one or both parents. It is important to note that typically the misalignment is not discernable by cursory observation and presents no cosmetic concerns to family or friends, but visual symptoms will be present such as poor reading skills. We want to emphasize that having a very small vertical phoria corrected is vital in helping a child's reading and learning abilities. This is due to the fact that many eye care professionals disregard all vertical imbalances except the very large ones, thus failing to help countless individuals. We routinely find that the correction of as little as ¼ prism diopter of vertical phoria in children results in a marked improvement of reading and comprehension ability at school.

Vertical phoria is a condition that results in disrupting a person's binocular vision (ability of the eyes to stay aligned and working together) and interferes in the maintaining fixation of both eyes on a target during any process that requires re-fixation; i.e, the eyes change from the end of one line down to the next line when reading. That is why a near vertical phoria will especially have a detrimental effect on children's reading ability, reading comprehension, and over all learning progress in school. This commonly results in a child having below average reading skills and falling behind in their class work.

A distance vertical phoria generally results in motion sickness and depth perception problems, which will impact a child's ability in such activities as baseball, softball, and other sports. Car sickness and sea sickness are common symptoms as well and is due to the disparity between visual inputs being different from vestibular input.

To better understand this visual condition, it is helpful to know what it is not. First, as stated before, it is not clearness of vision or visual acuity at distance and near (reading letters on an eye chart). The acuity chart tests the ability of a person to read a predetermined size of letters or numbers at a certain distance. That is why a routine vision screening at school, general family practice, or pediatrician doctor's office may detect some children's trouble seeing the distance eye chart and other more obvious vision conditions, but they will always miss other visual skills such as the inability of the child's eyes to achieve and maintain proper near focus, eye muscle co-ordination, horizontal and vertical eye coordination, as well as other vision skills that are absolutely fundamental in classroom work.

Therefore, it is important to repeat that a child may read 20/20 letters just fine on a screening test for distance vision but may have great difficulty with concentration and reading at near. That's why it is so important to have an exam by an eye care professional that will also check for binocular vision skills including vertical phoria around the time school starts each year. In a nutshell, good vision is so much more than reading a 20/20 line of letters on a wall chart.

Vertical phoria is not a function of how well the eyes are able to focus at near (known as accommodation), or with the eyes tracking a steadily moving object such as a penlight (called pursuits). Also, the range of eye muscle movement is not affected in the field of gazes to the left, right, up, or down. Convergence (ability of the eyes to turn inward to focus on a near object) is not the same. All these visual skills are important and vital to give your child the opportunity to do well in school.

Signs and symptoms will be discussed in more detail in the next chapter, but you should keep in mind that this condition, as a rule, is missed and goes undiagnosed even at many optometrist and ophthalmologist's eye exams due to the eye doctor not being more watchful for the signs and symptom of vertical phoria. That's why we call it the forgotten diagnosis.

We recommend that questions relating to a child's schoolwork and reading level should always be asked by all vision specialists at the time of the child's medical and the visual history prior to the actual eye exam testing.

Topics such as how the child is doing in school, trouble with reading, using a finger to help read on a line, using color sheets over print, tired eyes when reading, hating to read, car sickness, or headaches when reading should direct the eye doctor to evaluate for the presence of a vertical phoria.

If you think you or your child may have a vertical phoria due to the presence of symptoms discussed, how are you going to locate an optometrist or ophthalmologist who will check for the possibility of vertical phoria and appropriately prescribe to correct it? You need to find a local provider who is readily aware of vertical phoria symptoms and management. This can be done by phoning local eye doctors' offices and asking if they diagnose and treat binocular disorders of vision in children. The basic vision test for a child with reading problems should include, at a minimum, the following tests:

- Acuity: distance (clearness test on reading chart)
- Focus at near with evaluation of amount and flexibility
- Refraction (need for glasses)
- Eye convergence
- Eye pursuits
- Eye tracking
- Horizontal binocular alignment at distance and near
- Vertical binocular alignment at distance and near
- Evaluation of eye health

The above list is not to suggest that it is comprehensive or is the only visual test needed for all children. Other factors that always must be considered by the vision specialist include medical, behavioral, or neurological conditions that are important to consider in a child's capacity for excellent reading skills, cognitive function, and learning skills. It is best to have a coordinated team effort between professional disciplines such as optometrists, physicians, child psychologists or child psychiatrists, speech and language specialists, as well as vision perception therapists for children who continue to struggle in school with learning disabilities or social disabilities.

Let us be clear that having a vertical phoria diagnosed and corrected does not rule out other issues being present that are very real and need proper treatment to help a child in school. It has been our experience that the correction of any vertical phoria is all that is needed to help a child do extremely well in reading. It also may be true that other vision, emotional, motivational, psychiatric, and developmental problems will go hand in hand to help children with learning disabilities that need professional attention additionally.

We recommend a fully integrated approach between various specialties at an ealy age for children who are constantly struggling in school. A psycho-educational evaluation is the most comprehensive approach to explore multiple possible causes for a child's ongoing learning difficulty. Here is a partial list of factors that can directly impact a child's learning ability:

- Poor vision at distance and/or near. Possibly poor vision at near only
- Poor eye coordination and focusing
- Poor visual processing and comprehension
- Anxiety disorders
- Depression
- Poor self-esteem
- Parent-Parent conflicts
- Parent-Child conflicts
- Peer relationships
- Emotional trauma
- Hearing problems

- Child's IQ
- Teaching style
- Classroom environment

Now that you have a better understanding of what correct vision skills consist of and are aware of how it is one of the most indispensable foundations involved in learning, let's talk in the next chapter about what symptoms in particular you need to be aware of that may point to the presence of a vertical phoria.

CHAPTER 4

Symptoms of Vertical Phoria

What are the most common symptoms to be aware of with uncorrected vertical phoria? As described in the book's examples, individuals may relate their visual experiences in abstract terms such as trouble in school, being disruptive in class, headaches, eyes getting tired easily, or the inability to concentrate when reading. All these symptoms should make you and your eye doctor think of checking for the presence of a vertical phoria. Don't be surprised if you have to ask for the eye doctor to test for the presence of a vertical phoria. Now that you are aware that vision is more than being able to read the 20/20 line on the eye chart, your eye doctor needs to always ask more specific questions concerning visual perception and performance in school in addition to testing for refractive error and ruling out eye disease.

In our practice we like to ask such questions as how the child is doing in school at the beginning of the eye examination. This is especially true in children who are having difficulties in school academics, which the parents often do not relate to vision, many times because they have been told their child has 20/20 vision. Our office has devised a form with a checklist (included for your reference) which we have the patient or parent complete prior to exam. This helps to make us aware of any undiagnosed reading issues possibly related to a vertical phoria that needs to be corrected.

Let's review some of the most common symptoms of vertical phoria to use as a checklist:

- Person does not like to read in a moving car
- Person does not like to sit in the rear seat of a moving car
- Motion sickness
- Sea sickness
- Fear of heights
- Person loses their place while reading
- Person forgets what they read
- Skipping or re-reading lines
- Headaches and/or eye strain when reading
- Person tilts head to use one eye better when reading
- Person has an aversion to being spun around
- Person uses a finger to keep from losing place when reading
- Avoiding close work
- Rubbing the eyes when doing close visual tasks
- Avoiding a computer because the eyes hurt
- Receiving lower grades than usual
- Decreased or delayed reading comprehension
- Poor school performance in one or more subjects

As stated before, your first clue with young children is generally related to a history of poor school performance. Having children receive a comprehensive eye exam each year at the beginning of school would help ensure that any needed vision correction by prescription glasses or contact lenses, how the eyes are focusing at near for reading, and working together at distance and near viewing would eliminate many learning difficulties in schoolwork. Other eye conditions, medical conditions, and psychological factors must always be considered if a child continues to do poorly in school after a comprehensive eye examination results in normal findings.

A vertical phoria, when uncorrected, usually has a marked detrimental effect on a child's school performance and is an inherited trait in which one of the parents most likely will have similar symptoms as previously mentioned. Occasionally, vertical phoria will skip a generation and show up in grandchildren.

Interestingly, vertical phoria usually causes difficulty with schoolwork in males more than females. It seems that male children get frustrated faster and easier if they are having trouble reading or keeping up in class with their peers, resulting in restlessness and behavioral issues.

We often see children who can easily read the 20/20 line or our exam room distance acuity chart and near acuity chart, pass the entire basic vision test but are still doing poorly in school. These children are highly suspicious for having a vertical phoria or other binocular problem.

Unfortunately, we do not know how many of these children with undiagnosed vertical phoria have been wrongly labeled as learning disabled, dyslexic, ADHD, or ADD because they cannot sit still and concentrate on reading. These children are generally automatically prescribed psychoactive drugs and never referred to an eye specialist for an evaluation of their binocular function.

When children are corrected with appropriate prescription glasses to correct a vertical phoria, it is not uncommon for these children to excel dramatically in school right away. This works because a prism is prescribed to bend the light coming into the eye so as to produce the correct alignment of the visual axis of both eyes, so that they work and focus together instead of fighting each other when reading.

With a vertical phoria, some children may need additional special visual training to maximize their binocular function and comprehension. Your optometrist may refer you to another optometrist or other discipline that specializes in visual motor training and tasks targeted to overcome certain learning impediments. Some occupational therapists specialize in vision and binocular therapy that can help these children.

A recent study by the University of California San Diego Shiley Eye Center, which appears in the February issue of Archives of Ophthalmology, confirms that preschoolers with uncorrected vision issues have lower scores in development testing and success in school performance (the Beery-Buktenica Developmental Test of Visual-Motor Integration, also known as Developmental Test of Visual-Motor Integration or VMI, which tests visual-motor integration and visual construction skills). It identifies problems with visual perception, motor coordination, and visual-motor integration such as hand-eye coordination. Read more at: *http:// www. answers. com/topic/beery-buktenica-test-1#ixzz1XOYFeoiw.* But those scores improve significantly within six weeks when children are provided the correct prescription glasses to wear.

We would like to see all teachers and parents across our country recognize a child's reading or learning difficulty in school as a need to generate an appointment with an optometrist who is knowledgeable in the diagnosis and treatment of not only the most common visual disorders but who also evaluates for binocular problems including vertical phoria.

CHAPTER 5

Testing for Vertical Phoria

Now that you know of the symptoms related to vertical phoria, let's talk about how the eye doctor will clinically verify the diagnosis and measure any amount of phoria deviation for a corrective prescription at the doctor's office. The direction and amount of prism needed to align the visual axis of the eyes must be measured and quantified by your eye doctor. Prisms, as you may know, bend light and are prescribed to bend light to the proper alignment needed for the eyes. Your eye doctor may want to use several accepted exam methods of testing to be confident of the exact prism power, and direction will be needed to eliminate an individual's symptoms and achieve the best binocular results for the child.

The most important and most time consuming part of the management of vertical phoria depends on the proper detection and treatment based on the individual symptoms and all other clinical tests combined with psychological factors.

The eye doctor must be sure all other aspects of the eye exam, such as correction for nearsightedness, farsightedness, astigmatism, the eyes' ability to focus at near, ocular health, as well as other factors have been addressed first. At the time of the initial visit, your eye doctor must be asking the right questions, such as the ones listed in the previous chapter concerning school. At our office we have these questions located on our patient history form to alert us to any indication a child has a possible diagnosis of vertical phoria and is unaware of what is causing their difficulty with schoolwork.

After all other components of the vision examination have finished, your optometrist will perform some or all of the following tests and, if required, other tests that are not part of the basic eye exam. Special visual system testing will confirm and precisely determine what prism to prescribe. Your eye doctor should be happy to explain how these tests work during the exam.

But don't worry about the name of these tests or how they work; what is important is the outcome with improved reading and academic achievement. Testing includes but is not limited to the following methods:

- Von Graffe Test, with or without color filters at distance and near

- Maddox Rod Test at distance and near

- Cover Test at distance and near

- Titmus Vision Screening Tester

- Fixation Disparity Test

Once the new glasses with proper prescription prism are worn for a few days or weeks, almost all parents and children report immediate improvement in reading skills and school grades. Occasionally a small adjustment in the prism may be needed after the prescription glasses have been worn for a few weeks. Make sure you are given another appointment with the eye doctor in three or four weeks after the dispensing of corrective lenses for vertical phoria to ensure the symptoms are eliminated and for a check in alignment of the eyes with the new prescription glasses.

CHAPTER 6

Especially for Parents

Most people may not be aware that according to the medical community guidelines, a diagnosis of ADHD, DSM-IV, implies the presence of hyperactive-impulsive or inattentive symptoms that caused impairment and were present before age seven. The symptoms must cause clinically significant impairment; e.g., in social, academic, or occupational functioning, and be present in two or more settings; e.g., school (or work), and at home. The symptoms must not be better accounted for by another mental disorder. For the inattentive type, at least six of the following symptoms must have persisted for at least six months: lack of attention to details/careless mistakes, lack of sustained attention, poor listener, failure to follow through on tasks, poor organization, avoids tasks requiring sustained mental effort, loses things, easily distracted, forgetful.

Doesn't the above definition sound exactly like a child who is having difficulty in school due to an uncorrected vision problem such as a vertical phoria and cannot sit still or pay attention? Please make a special note than an evaluation for vision-related disorders is never considered in the medical definition and diagnosing of ADHD. This is because the medical evaluation for ADD and ADHD does not include a baseline complete evaluation of vision and visual perception skills as part of the diagnosis protocol, and also why prescription psychoactive drugs are so quickly given automatically by most medical practitioners to calm children down.

Unfortunately, the majority of pediatric physicians who are quick to prescribe drugs for these children do not have the education and training background to detect and refer a child to an optometrist for a visual examination, which would rule out one or more of the binocular vision or perception disorders discussed in this book that result in poor school performance, but instead are trained to look for mental and medical disorders.

Again, this is why prescription drugs for children with these symptoms are commonly the preferred treatment of choice within the medical profession and results in the children being drugged so as not to be disruptive in class. This is extremely unfortunate for so many children and their parents.

Separately or combined, accommodative disorders, convergence insufficiency, divergence excess, and a vertical phoria can result in symptoms that would be consistent with a child being diagnosed as ADHD, dyslexic, or slow learning.

Drugs may or may not be necessary for a child with learning problems, but should not be the first choice in management. Instead, children falling behind in school should have a referral to an eye professional with knowledge of behavioral and development vision. This would be a much more appropriate first choice to establish a baseline for detection and correction of any visual functions and vision abilities prior to any other therapy being provided for a child with normal intelligence.

According to an article published in July 2009 by Joel Zaba, MA, OD, one in four school children have had a vision problem and it is one of the most prevalent handicapping conditions in childhood. Research has shown that only 10 percent of children aged nine to fifteen who needed prescription glasses actually had them.

Even more alarming is that when children are identified with vision problems, during vision screenings at school or a pediatrician's office, only 33-60 percent receive a needed full eye exam or vision correction. This does not speak well of parents looking out for the welfare of their children. We urge you to make yearly eye exam appointments for yourself and especially your children to ensure any vision problems or changes in a prescription are identified and corrected at the beginning of each school year.

Everyone should understand that the failure of parents to get their children the vision help they need early in their academic endeavors directly affects issues such as childhood development, learning ability, self-esteem, social-emotional interactive behavior, high school dropout rates, and eventually juvenile delinquency.

Having and sharing the knowledge in this book with all parents, educational professionals, and healthcare professionals nationwide will keep millions of children from doing poorly in school, being improperly labeled, and being placed on psychoactive prescription drugs or therapy programs that may not be needed at all.

One of the first steps in a child's evaluation for learning difficulties should always be a thorough vision evaluation by an eye professional who is educated and trained to understand these visual conditions, and always checking, in addition to all the routine vision tests, for the presence of binocular trouble such as vertical phoria in children that are having difficulty with schoolwork. Failure to have a complete eye test for vision disorders by a vision specialist, including vertical phoria, in children starting school often leads to trouble in their reading ability and schoolwork performance. This results not only in a waste of educational funding resources, a higher juvenile a delinquency rate, and more career criminals in our society, but also an unnecessary failure in cultivating a child's intelligence, academic achievement, potential standard of living, and career potential.

The fact of the matter is that this is an enormous national issue that affects all Americans in terms of dollars wasted on methods that do not address root causes of poor school performance and loss of productivity of our future adult citizens.

Presently the solution starts at home with you, the parent or legal guardian, making a vision examination appointment with the correct vision specialist every year around the time school starts. As of the writing of this, Kentucky, Missouri, and Illinois are the only states that have laws requiring mandatory eye examinations for children prior to entering school and a federal bill has been introduced in the Senate that would provide funding to establish a federal grant program focusing on treatment to bolster children's vision initiatives in the states and encourage children's vision partnerships with non-profit entities. Hopefully, one day all children will be required to take and have access to a comprehensive vision examination prior to entering school for not only their future but our country's future. This will no doubt require a large grassroots effort across the country to get state and federal governments to fully address this important matter in a thorough and effective manner.

CHAPTER 7

Summary for Family Reading Together

You are now aware that in the school environment there are many visual, social, psychological, and medically related conditions that can affect children's reading, learning, and comprehension skills. Most optometrist and ophthalmologists agree to have a child's first eye exam no later than the fourth year, followed by yearly visits to the eye doctor. Don't forget, school vision screenings and pediatrician screenings are not intended to substitute for the eye doctor's yearly exams, nor will they uncover any but the most apparent vision problems.

This book is intended to help educate the public not only on how essential proper vision and visual skills are to learning, but also about a specific binocular visual condition (vertical phoria) that is most often forgotten by eye specialists when presented with a person complaining of reading of learning difficulties. We have focused our discussion on *vertical phoria*, one of several binocular eye disorders associated with poor school performance, in order to bring this correctible visual anomaly to the public's attention in hopes of helping as many children as possible across our country from being incorrectly labeled as learning disabled or ADHD, having to take unnecessary medication, and to help them achieve their full potential in life.

Our goal is that the public will become more aware of the need for early comprehensive vision exams for children prior to entering school, with special emphasis on children having trouble with school-work, possibly due to vertical phoria or other binocular disorders, along with where to seek help for the proper diagnosis and treatment. This information is especially important for parents who have children who are already struggling with learning and keeping up with schoolwork.

Remember, vertical phoria is a visual anomaly that is very often overlooked and forgotten by many, if not most, eye practitioners at the time of an eye examination in determining the cause and treatment of a person complaining of any or all of the following: headaches, tired eyes, poor concentration, poor reading skills, poor school performance and motion sickness. Vertical phoria directly hinders reading and learning skills, which is especially important in school-aged children and college students.

Important points for the parent to know and remember are as follows:

1. *Vertical phoria is not dyslexia.* Dyslexia simply means trouble reading and there are seven types of dyslexia. Vertical phoria can be present with or without dyslexia. Vertical phoria can exacerbate dyslexia symptoms. Vision, ocular, and binocular baseline tests should be done first in all children having trouble with schoolwork prior to a diagnosis of dyslexia.

2. *Vertical phoria is not an attention deficit disorder.* Vertical phoria can be present with or without attention deficit disorder. Vertical phoria can dramatically aggravate a child's attention deficit disorder. Rule out vision problems first.

3. *Vertical phoria is not an eye tracking problem* that involves small, continuous, and smooth eye movements to follow a target or read across a page.

4. *Vertical phoria is not a static fixation problem,* but has to do with dynamic fixation (re-fixation) as with changing eye positions on different objects or locations on a page. The failure of a child's eyes to re-fixate automatically when reading down to the next line of print results in loss of place and a break in concentration. This is why using a finger or book marker helps these children stay on line.

5. *Vertical phoria is not a convergence insufficiency disorder,* which involves the inability to bring the eyes together in the horizontal plane for close tasks, such as reading, due to weak eye muscles.

6. *Vertical phoria is not a divergence excess disorder,* which is when the eyes want to separate in the horizontal plane due to weak eye muscles.

7. *Vertical phoria is not an accommodation disorder,* involving the eyes focusing like a camera to near objects versus distance objects.

These last three anomalies are all binocular problems involving the eyes working together and directly impacts a child's close vision tasks such as reading ability and reading comprehension.

1. Convergence insufficiency

2. Divergence excess

3. Accommodative disorders

Now you know that vertical phoria affects a child's reading ability by affecting his inability to fixate and concentrate easily with both eyes. This is why the presence of a vertical phoria interferes with a child's reading ability, comprehension, and learning. You will notice that the symptoms may be overlapping between the four binocular conditions: convergence insufficiency, divergence excess, accommodative disorders, along with vertical phoria. Only vision specialists such as an optometrist, who is familiar with these conditions, will be able to make the proper diagnosis and prescribe the correct treatment.

This book emphasizes vertical phoria information and understanding because it is very common in the population and is correctable with prism in prescription glasses. It is estimated that one out of four children have learning disorders in the U.S., and as many as one in seven children have a vertical phoria! We are talking about millions of children in our country who are treatable yet go undiagnosed and untreated every year.

As stated earlier, vertical phoria is by far one of the most missed or forgotten diagnoses in young people simply because it is overlooked by the very professionals trained to help individuals with learning difficulties.

Parents, teachers, reading instructors, and general physicians can all help by referring children to have a full vision evaluation (being sure to include binocular skills testing) at the beginning of each school year. By knowing there are certain symptoms to watch for and bringing these symptoms to the attention of your eye doctor, he will help ensure there are no uncorrected visual irregularities.

So, what does a parent do? First take another look at the provided symptoms checklist for vertical phoria. Is your child struggling in school? Does your child have some or all of these symptoms? Next, schedule an appointment with an optometrist who is familiar with this condition. He or she may call themselves *behavioral or developmental optometrists* and indicate they do vision therapy. Some other eye professions are aware of this condition, but you will get the most thorough help from a behavioral or developmental optometrist. These doctors have spent four years in an optometry professional school training program and then specialize in behavioral and developmental vision issues. They have the most knowledge and office equipment to properly diagnosis and treat your child for any of the mentioned binocular vision problems.

When you take your child to any optometrist to make sure their eyes are seeing 20/20, focusing accurately, and working together properly for optimal learning ability, make sure the optometrist is familiar and experienced with managing these discussed conditions. They will run a battery of tests to evaluate your child's visual acuity, accommodative ability, and binocular skills, as well as the health of the eyes, to rule out any disease or disorders affecting vision. Be sure to copy and fill out the symptoms checklist for vertical phoria found in this book to take with you to your optometrist.

Be comforted to know that the conditions we are talking about in this book are not disease-related but have to do with skills and developmental weakness in the visual system that relate to the level of cognitive abilities and ease of learning. They may be corrected with eye exercises, glasses with a regarding Rx, glasses with prism Rx, glasses with reading and prism Rx, or a combination of the above depending on the diagnosis. Results are usually dramatic and noted quickly by parents as their child's reading skills and levels of achievement in school improve rapidly.

Correction with eye exercises is appropriate for certain vision problems and involves either an in-office program of multiple visits of thirty to sixty minutes per session, or purchasing a vision therapy kit for home training. The cost involved will vary depending on the type of therapy, length of therapy, in-office sessions, or if a home training kit is chosen. Expect to invest $330 or more for a home training kit and $600 or more for training sessions in a doctor's office, or with an occupational therapist. Each office sets their office fees on the required therapy prescribed and the time required.

Correction using prescription glasses for vertical phoria involves prisms to redirect where the light strikes the retina. If a bifocal prescription for other than vertical phoria is needed, ask the doctor if a progressive lens will work in your child's situation. Make sure another appointment is made in a few weeks to evaluate if the treatment is as effective as expected or if modification of treatment is needed.

Now you know how important it is to keep yearly vision exam appointments that are comprehensive in scope for your children and not rely on screenings at the school or pediatrician's office. Your child's future success in school and life is truly in your hands!

APPENDIX

Vision Vocabulary

Amblyopia ("lazy eye"): A visual defect that affects approximately two or three out of every one hundred children in the United States. Amblyopia involves lowered visual acuity (clarity) and/or poor muscle control in one eye. The result is often a loss of stereoscopic vision and binocular depth perception. Vision therapy can benefit this condition, but early detection is very important. For many years, it was thought that amblyopia (lazy eye) was only amenable to treatment during the *critical period*. This is the period up to age seven or eight years. Current research has conclusively demonstrated that effective treatment can take place at any age, but the length of the treatment period increases dramatically the longer the condition has existed prior to treatment. Research has also demonstrated that patients with amblyopia are more likely to sustain injuries resulting in the loss of their good eye than individuals with two good eyes. There are many reasons that early childhood eye examinations are essential.

Binocular: Of or involving both eyes at once working together.

Binocular depth perception: A result of successful stereo vision; the ability to visually perceive three dimensional space; the ability to visually judge relative distances between objects; a visual skill that aids accurate movement in three-dimensional space.

Binocular vision: Vision as a result of both eyes working as a team; when both eyes work together smoothly, accurately, equally, and simultaneously.

Binocular vision disability: A visual defect in which the two eyes fail to work together as a coordinated team, resulting in a partial or total loss of binocular depth perception and stereoscopic vision. At least 12 percent of the population has some type of binocular vision disability. Amblyopia and strabismus are the most commonly known types of binocular vision disabilities.

Developmental/behavioral optometry: A branch of optometry which specializes in the practice of vision therapy to enhance and/or correct visual performance skills. Behavioral optometrists (also called developmental optometrists) will consider how environmental, nutritional, and/or behavioral factors effect visual capability and prescribe or recommend corrective action.

Ophthalmologist: A doctor of ophthalmology is an eye specialist trained specifically in the knowledge and skills for eye surgery, treating eye diseases, and injuries to the eye and surrounding area.

Optometrist: A doctor of optometry is an eye/vision specialist trained in the knowledge and skills for treating certain eye diseases and injuries, examining and treating any reduced visual performance skills, prescribing glasses and contact lenses, fitting special optical devices vision-impaired individuals, and performing vision therapy.

Orthoptics: The eye muscle training techniques or orthoptics are included within vision therapy. Orthoptics specifically treat eye teaming skills and visual acuity and do not treat other visual dysfunctions which are addressed by vision therapy procedures. Orthoptics first became popular in Europe in the 1900s. David Wells, MD, an ophthalmologist at Boston University, is credited with introducing orthoptics to the U.S. in 1912. Orthoptics are still practiced by a small percentage of optometrists, ophthalmologists, and orthoptic therapists.

Stereo vision (stereopsis or stereoscopic vision): A byproduct of good binocular vision; vision wherein the separate images from two eyes are successfully combined into one three-dimensional image in the brain.

Strabismus ("crossed eye", "wall eye", "wandering eye", esotropia, exotropia, hyperphoria): Affects approximately four out of every one hundred children in the United States. It is a visual defect in which the two eyes point in different directions. One eye may turn either in, out, up, or down while the other eye aims straight ahead. Due to this condition, both eyes do not always aim simultaneously at the same object. This results in a partial or total loss of stereo vision and binocular depth perception. The eye turns may be visible at all times or may come and go. In some cases, the eye misalignments are not obvious to the untrained observer.

Vision: The act of perceiving and interpreting visual information with the eyes, mind, and body.

Vision therapy (also known as "vision training"): Therapy involving exercises which are aimed at improving visual skills such as, eye teaming, binocular coordination and depth perception, focusing, acuity (clarity of sight), and "hand-eye" or "vision-body" coordination. Vision therapy can involve a variety of procedures to correct neurophysiological or neurosensory visual dysfunctions.

Patient Success Stories

I have many more stories of successful kids. Here are just two:

Grace was six years old when she first saw us. She was sent by a child neuropsychologist for evaluation of visual, spatial, and reading problems. It was an over two-hour drive to our office. She was very typical of our patient base. She had great distance vision and had been seen by several eye doctors, each telling her that her problems were not visual. Her parents were highly educated and felt her constant eye rubbing and dislike for reading suggested some visual issue. They were right. Grace had a large vertical eye misalignment plus another visual skills issue called accommodative insufficiency. To help correct her issues, she needed a prism to correct the vertical phoria and bifocal reading lenses to ease the accommodative insufficiency. The results were remarkable and the follow-ups were encouraging. I do expect her to no longer need the glasses in a few years.

Dakota had been sent to us by his school, a bright ten-year-old male who was struggling to keep up with his class in reading and general homework. He had great vision and was told by his doctor that vision was not the issue. He had been put on ADD medication. We did a full binocular evaluation. He had two main visual skills problems, vertical eye misalignment and the ability to change visual focus. We prescribed reading glasses and the results were immediate. The school called in three weeks to say how much improvement they had seen. Dakota was smiling a lot at his follow-up; his mom was so happy she was crying. The beauty is after the glasses and the visual training he should be out of the glasses in two years.

I now want to give examples of adults. Adults express their complaints differently than children. They complain more of headaches and eye strain. They have usually developed some compensation skills to help overcome the reading comprehension issue caused by the lack of binocular skills. However, they still struggle with reading and eye strain.

Vickie is a forty-three-year-old female with complaints of migraines and eye strain even with her bifocal glasses. She was recommended to us by a friend. Her complaints were that she would lose her place often and quit reading after only ten minutes. After the binocular exam, we diagnosed her as having visual misalignment. We made her glasses with prism. This resolved the reading issue and greatly reduced the occurrence of her migraines.

Another adult is **Jessica**, a twenty-four-year-old female with 20/20 distance vision. She had done well in school, but felt she had to work much harder than her fellow students. Once again after the binocular exam we found she had eye misalignment and a visual focusing problem. We treated her with a reading prescription, which included both prism and power. The patient called back in less than two weeks saying how much easier it was to read.

Another adult, **Paula** was sent to us by a friend. She was in for a medical eye condition. However, during the questioning phase of the exam she reported headaches with regard to losing her place. After evaluating her, we prescribed reading glasses with a prism. She was very excited with the ability to read smoothly without losing her place.

Checklist for Parents

Vertical Phoria Symptoms:

- Dislikes reading in a moving car
- Dislikes riding in the back seat of a moving car, prefers front
- Dislikes being spun around
- Fear of heights
- Skip lines while reading
- Re-reading lines
- Loses place while reading
- Using a finger to stay on a line while reading
- Turn or tilting the head to favor one eye
- Poor comprehension, can't remember what was read
- Words jumble or move on the page
- Eyestrain while reading
- Avoiding close work
- Motion sickness
- Sea sickness
- Receiving lower grades than usual
- Decreased or delayed reading comprehension
- Poor school performance in one or more subjects

Endnotes

Cott, Allan, MD, *Help for Your Learning-Disabled Child,*
(New York: Crown Publishing, 1985).

Kline, Carl L., MD, with Carolyn Lacey Kline, "The Epidemic of
Reading Disabilities," www.readingstore.com.

Moffitt, Terrie, "Adolescence-limited and Life-course-persistent
Antisocial Behavior: A Developmental Taxonomy," American
Psychology Association, *Psychological Review*, Vol. 100, 1993,
http://psycnet.apa.org/index.cfm?fa=buy.optionToBuy&id=19
94-05949-001.

Hogenson, Dennis, "Reading Failure and Juvenile
Delinquency," *Annals of Dyslexia*, Volume 24, No. 1.

National Center for Education Statistics, Literacy in Everyday
Life: Results from the 2003 National Assessment of Adult
Literacy. NCES 2007-490, Available from ED Pubs., P.O. Box
1398, Jessup, MD 20794-1398,
http://nces.ed.gov/help/orderinfo.asp.

Reading Connections, 122 North Elm Street, Suite 520,
Greensboro, NC 27401 (2011), http://www.readingcon-
nections.org/program-literacy-facts.asp.

Brunner, M.S., "Reduced Recidivism and Increased Employment Opportunity through Research-Based Reading Instruction"; Office of Juvenile Justice and Delinquency Prevention, U.S. Department of Justice, Washington, D.C., January 1993.

Granet, David B.; Gomi, Cintia F; Ventura, Ricardo; Miller-Scholte, Andrea, "The Relationship between Convergence Insufficiency and ADHD," Strabismus, 13:4, 2005.

National PTA, *Learning Related Vision Problems Education and Evaluation,* Resolution adopted at National PTA Convention, June 26-29, 1999, Portland, OR.

Zaba, Joel. "Many Children Today Lack Good Vision Care," *Ophthalmology Times,* August 26, 2009, http://optometrytimes.modernmedicine.com/children.

Resources

Snow, C.E.; Burns, S.M.; and Griffin, P., Eds, *Preventing Reading Difficulties in Young Children*, Washington, D.C.: National Academy Press, 1998.

Zaba, Joel N., "Children's Vision Care in the 21st Century and Its Impact on Education, Literacy, Social Issues, and the Workplace: A Call to Action," *Journal of Behavioral Optometry*, Vol. 22, Issue 2, 2011.

Flores, J. Robert, "Risk and Protective Factors," April, 2003. http://www.ncjrs.gov/pdffiles1/ojjdp/193409.pdf

Hinds, Marian, "Illiteracy and Violence: Confusion about Cause and Effect," 2002, www.readingstore.com

National Assessment of Adult Literacy, 2003, "Literacy in Everyday Life: Results from the 2003 National Assessment of Adult Literacy," http://nces.ed.gov/naa//

Centers for Disease Control and Prevention, "Visual Impairment and Use of Eye-care Services and Protective Eyewear among Children – United States," 2002, *Morbidity and Mortality Weekly* Report, 2005.

Press, Dr. Leonard J., OD, FAAO, "Students with Persistent Problems – The Visual Connection," *School Nurse News*, September, 2000.

www.ingramcontent.com/pod-product-compliance
Lightning Source LLC
Chambersburg PA
CBHW041224050726
47599CB00001B/66